YOUR KNOWLEDGE HAS VALUE

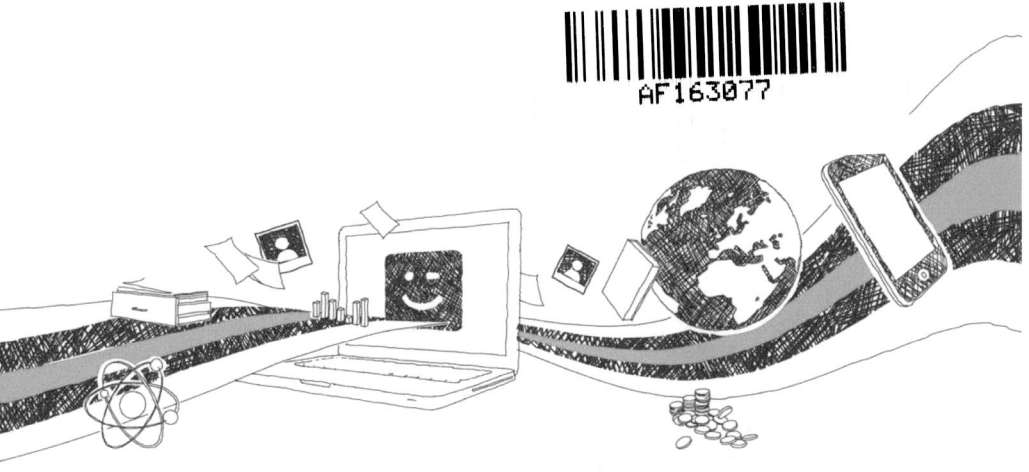

- We will publish your bachelor's and master's thesis, essays and papers

- Your own eBook and book - sold worldwide in all relevant shops

- Earn money with each sale

Upload your text at www.GRIN.com and publish for free

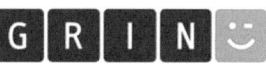

Bibliographic information published by the German National Library:

The German National Library lists this publication in the National Bibliography; detailed bibliographic data are available on the Internet at http://dnb.dnb.de .

This book is copyright material and must not be copied, reproduced, transferred, distributed, leased, licensed or publicly performed or used in any way except as specifically permitted in writing by the publishers, as allowed under the terms and conditions under which it was purchased or as strictly permitted by applicable copyright law. Any unauthorized distribution or use of this text may be a direct infringement of the author s and publisher s rights and those responsible may be liable in law accordingly.

Imprint:

Copyright © 2017 GRIN Verlag, Open Publishing GmbH
Print and binding: Books on Demand GmbH, Norderstedt Germany
ISBN: 9783668597297

This book at GRIN:

https://www.grin.com/document/384976

Patrick Kimuyu

Pulmonary Embolism. Prevalence, Diagnosis and Management

GRIN Publishing

GRIN - Your knowledge has value

Since its foundation in 1998, GRIN has specialized in publishing academic texts by students, college teachers and other academics as e-book and printed book. The website www.grin.com is an ideal platform for presenting term papers, final papers, scientific essays, dissertations and specialist books.

Visit us on the internet:

http://www.grin.com/

http://www.facebook.com/grincom

http://www.twitter.com/grin_com

Pulmonary Embolism: Prevalence, Diagnosis and Management

Name: Patrick Kimuyu

Introduction

Pulmonary embolism is usually a life-threatening condition that occurs due to blockage of the main artery carrying blood to the lungs. This blockage is caused by a blood clot that is carried in the bloodstream to the lung, primarily from the leg following deep vein thrombosis. From a primary care perspective, pulmonary embolism is not considered as a disease with its etiology. Rather, it arises as a complication of a number of conditions that cause venous thrombosis such as deep vein thrombosis, pregnancy and postoperative complications (Ouellette, 2015). This literature review focuses on evaluating current evidence based guidelines for diagnosis and management of pulmonary embolism.

Incidence and Prevalence

Epidemiological trends of pulmonary embolism vary from country to country and among different populations. In the United States, pulmonary embolism has become a public health problem due to its high prevalence and incidence. Currently, about 250,000 new cases of pulmonary embolism occur annually. This accounts for an incidence of 1 person per every 1000 people in the US. Clinical data indicate that pulmonary embolism accounts for 200,000 deaths, annually. Three decades ago, the prevalence of the disease was 6%, but clinical interventions and improved diagnosis has lowered it to 2% (Abbas & Mitchell, 2010).

Pathophysiology

From the nursing perspective, the physiology of pulmonary embolism can be explained through its main physiological consequences in the body. Ordinarily, pulmonary embolism is associated with hemodynamic and respiratory consequences. Regarding respiratory consequences, this condition caused death of alveoli leading to hyperventilation and hypoxemia. The principle mechanism of hypoxemia is attributable to reduced cardiac output, ventilation-perfusion mismatch, intracardiac shunt, primarily through foreman ovale, and intrapulmonary shunts. On the other hand, hemodynamic consequences are attributable to pulmonary vascular resistance that is caused by the decrease of pulmonary vascular bed. This resistance increases afterloads in the right ventricle and this might cause ventricular failure. It also involves pulmonary arterial constriction due to reflex and humoral mechanisms (Ouellette, 2015).

Clinical Implications of Pulmonary Embolism

In practice, pulmonary embolism has significant clinical implications. Foremost, the disease exhibits difficulties in diagnosis and its signs and symptoms are similar to those presented by other conditions such as chronic heart failure and COPD. On the other hand, it is a life-threatening condition that causes damage to the lungs and other vital organs. In most cases, failure to provide early clinical interventions leads to lung damage. This may cause pulmonary hypertension and failure of vital organs including the heart due to lack of oxygen supply. Therefore, it is apparent that pulmonary embolism requires appropriate clinical interventions, in order to minimize its related fatalities and morbidity.

Clinical Evidence-based Guidelines

In the past, most cases of pulmonary embolism were hardly noticed due to misdiagnosis. However, this challenge has been solved through the development of appropriate clinical evidence-based guidelines to aid diagnosis. In practice, probability testing guidelines and the rule-out criteria has become the mainstay in diagnosis of pulmonary embolism. The Wells Score and the Geneva Score are used to predict clinical probability, whereas the PERC (pulmonary embolism rule-out criteria) applies in the ruling out the risk of pulmonary embolism.

Wells Score clinical probability is based on suspected cases of deep vein thrombosis or its history, tachycardia, malignancy, hemoptysis, and immobilization. Based on Wells Score, a score of higher than 6.0 (59%) is considered as high probability, 2.0 to 6.0 (29%) is moderate, whereas less than 2.0 (15%) indicates low probability. Alternatively, a score greater than 4.0 indicates likelihood of pulmonary embolism so imaging is considered, whereas a score less than 4.0 indicates its unlikelihood, thus requiring D-dimer test for rule out. On the other hand, diagnostic testing that shows SaO_2 of less than 95% indicates low risk of pulmonary embolism, whereas any percentage above 95% is considered a high risk category.

Diagnostic Tests

Currently, there are several diagnostic tests for pulmonary embolism. The main tests include blood tests, imaging, electrocardiogram (ECG), and echocardiography. Blood tests are meant to identify any abnormality in the levels of various blood components or abnormal organ functions. The most commonly used blood tests are D-dimer, full blood count, blood coagulation tests (TT, PT and aPTT), liver enzymes test (LFT), renal function test, electrolytes test, and erythrocyte sedimentation rate (ESR).

D-dimer is considered as the primary test in patients with low and moderate probability of pulmonary embolism. A negative D-dimer test, in which results are based on the cut-off of 500ug/L, indicates the absence of pulmonary embolism (Schouten et al., 2013). However, suspicion of pulmonary embolism requires the other secondary blood tests.

On the other hand, imaging is recommended for patients with high probability of pulmonary embolism. In most cases, CT pulmonary angiography is used to identify changes in the lungs. Similarly, electrocardiogram is done to determine whether myocardial infarctions are the causes of chest pain. Some of the key diagnostic features of ECG related to pulmonary embolism include sinus tachycardia, blockage in the right bundle branch and right axis deviation.

Another useful diagnostic tool is echocardiography which is meant to evaluate thrombolysis, especially in patients with sub-massive and massive pulmonary embolism. This test identifies any dysfunction of the heart, especially the right compartment including obstruction in the right ventricle and pulmonary artery. Overall, echocardiography evaluates any deviation from the McConnell's sign, the normal appearance of the right ventricle.

Treatment/management

From the nursing perspective, clinical interventions are aimed at addressing the consequences associated with pulmonary embolism. The key management approaches include anticoagulant therapy, thrombolytic therapy and surgery.

It is recommended that all patients with suspected pulmonary embolism, as well as deep vein thrombosis should be placed on full anticoagulation, immediately without any delay owing to diagnostic investigations (Guyatt, Akl, Crowther, Gutterman & Schunemann, 2012). This therapy is aimed at preventing further formation of blood clots, and it is provide on long-term basis to prevent recurrence of the disease. Some of the medications used in the anticoagulant therapy include warfarin, fondaparinux, factor Xa inhibitors, and low-molecular-weight and unfractionated heparin.

On the other hand, thrombolytic therapy is recommended for patients experiencing acute pulmonary embolism, especially those with low bleeding risk. It is ideal for patients whose systolic blood pressure ranges below 90mmHg under hypotension conditions (Guyatt, Akl, Crowther, Gutterman & Schunemann, 2012). Some of the commonly used thrombotic agents include streptokinase, reteplase, alteplase, and urokinase.

Management of pulmonary embolism may require surgical options which are aimed at removing blood clots. The main surgical management options are the placement of vena cave filters and catheter embolectomy.

Follow-up Care

During the management of pulmonary embolism, patient education and follow-up care serve as paramount intervention approaches. Ideally, patient education enhances the patient's compliance to the treatment regimen. Of prime importance to patient's education is informing the patient of the complications associated with some of the drugs, primarily bleeding that occurs due interactions between heparin and warfarin with other drugs (Ouellette, 2015).

It is also important to provide follow-up care to patients with pulmonary embolism after treatment, in order to enhance recovery, and prevent recurrence. For instance, patients can be advised to wear compression stockings to prevent the formation of blood clots in the legs. It is also worth engaging the patient in regular leg exercise (Krans, 2015).

Prognosis

Prognosis of pulmonary embolism is based on two principal factors. The first factor is the appropriate diagnosis and management, whereas the second factor that determine prognosis of this condition is the underlying disease condition. Mortality for pulmonary embolism is usually reduced through anticoagulant treatment. Clinical studies show that mortality among patients with massive pulmonary embolism ranges from 30% to 60%. In most cases, high mortality rates of pulmonary embolism are indicated by elevated levels of natriuretic peptides and plasma lactate levels exceeding 2mmol/L. other significant prognosis factors include right-sided ventricular dysfunction, hypotension and injury markers (Vanni et al., 2013).

Differential Diagnosis

Presentation of pulmonary diagnosis is usually similar to that of other conditions. Therefore, differential diagnosis is necessary in confirming or excluding diagnosis of the disease. Differential diagnosis aims at screening for conditions such as occult neoplasm, lupus anticoagulant, connective tissue disorders, antithrombin III deficiency, and protein S or protein C deficiency.

Conclusion

Conclusively, pulmonary embolism is considered as a significant challenge to primary care. Epidemiological trends of the condition reveal that there are variations across the international demographics. In the US, incidence and prevalence of pulmonary embolism are relatively high. However, appropriate diagnosis and management approaches have led to the improvement of patients' outcome. For instance, international diagnostic guidelines such as the Well score, Geneva score and PERC which are used in probability testing serve as useful diagnostic algorithms. On the other hand, management approaches such as the anticoagulant therapy, thrombolytic therapy and surgical interventions play key roles in reducing pulmonary embolism related mortality.

Future Recommendation

Despite the success achieved in addressing pulmonary embolism, there are several issues that seem to impair the provision of primary care. Therefore, the following recommendations appear relevant in improving the diagnosis and management pulmonary embolism. First, there is need to define the most appropriate protocol for the interpretation of probability testing. Currently, physicians' interpretations are based on either the traditional or alternative interpretation approaches. This appears to compromise consistency in the clinical practice, primarily in relation to pulmonary embolism. Second, it is worth integrating home care into the management plan of pulmonary embolism. This will reduce treatment related complications and enhance patient's compliance to treatment regimen.

References

Abbas, K., & Mitchell, F. (2010). *Basic Pathology*. New Delhi, India: Elsevier.

Guyatt, G., Akl, E., Crowther, M., Gutterman, D., & Schunemann, H. (2012). Executive Summary: Antithrombotic therapy and prevention of thrombosis, 9th ed: American College of Chest Physicians evidence-based clinical practice guidelines. *Chest*, 141(2), 7S-47S.

Krans, B. (2015). *Pulmonary embolism*. Retrieved from http://www.healthline.com/health/pulmonary-embolus#Overview1

Ouellette, D. (2015). *Pulmonary embolism*. Retrieved from http://emedicine.medscape.com/article/300901-overview#showall

Schouten, H., Geersing, G., Koek, H., Zuithoff, N., Janssen, K., Douma, R., van Delden, J., Moons, K., & Reitsma, J. (2013). Diagnostic accuracy of conventional or age adjusted D-dimer cut-off values in older patients with suspected venous thromboembolism: systematic review and meta-analysis. *BMJ (Clinical Research ed.)*, 346: f2492. doi:10.1136/bmj.f2492.

Vanni, S., Viviani, G., Baioni, M., Pepe, G., Nazerian, P., & Socci, F. (2013). Prognostic value of plasma lactate levels among patients with acute pulmonary embolism: the thrombo-embolism lactate outcome study. *Ann Emerg Med.*, 61(3), 330-8.

YOUR KNOWLEDGE HAS VALUE

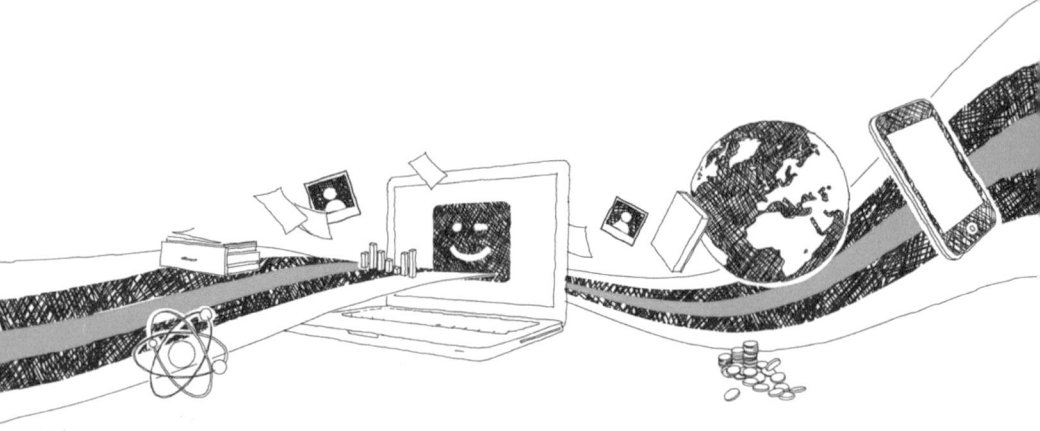

- We will publish your bachelor's and master's thesis, essays and papers

- Your own eBook and book - sold worldwide in all relevant shops

- Earn money with each sale

Upload your text at www.GRIN.com
and publish for free

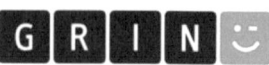